# EasyTerms™
# Terminology Guidebook
# for Nutrition

Copyright 2009, Ed Creager

This edition of EasyTerms is one in a series of simple-to-use, college-level terminology guidebooks.

Although these guidebooks were originally intended for college students, many High School students will also find them helpful as they prepare for college.

Other topics covered in existing or forthcoming editions:

- Anatomy & Physiology (Human)
- Biochemistry
- Biology
- Botany
- Business Management
- Cell Biology

- Ecology
- Genetics
- Microbiology
- Nursing
- Psychology
- Zoology

EasyTerms can help support your educational advancement and can boost the vocabulary of almost anyone who reads it.

For more information on these and other publications, please visit the author's site:

## www.edcreager.blogspot.com

and please note the author's "signature book" entitled,

## "The Money-Saving Idea Book: Inside Tips for Starving, Students, Frugal Seniors and Every Financial Survivor."

("The Money-Saving Idea Book" © and ™, Ed Creager, 2009.)

# Foreword

This Nutrition edition is a simple-to-use, college-level* terminology guidebook and is part of the EasyTerms reference series. In the book, terms are arranged alphabetically within appropriate topic areas. The complete index makes it easy to find any term and its definition.

* These books can also help High School students prepare so that, before they attend college, they'll already know a considerable amount of the terminology they'll need.

A substantial number of the terms defined here have additional definitions outside the scope of the subject being covered. More general definitions and additional meanings, if sought, are to be found in less specialized publications such as dictionaries and encyclopedias.

Please check the website of the author...

**www.edcreager.blogspot.com**

for more information on other available books.

To buy the Biology edition of EasyTerms and receive a Preferred Customer discount of 25%, please go to www.tinyurl.com/bookonbiology, click on "Add to Cart," and enter the **discount code "AAHN8EQH"** during check-out.

To save 25% on the Human Anatomy and Physiology edition, go to www.tinyurl.com/bookonanatomy, click on "Add to Cart," and enter the **discount code "M2LHBMP7"** during check-out.

Important Notice:

# EasyTerms™
## Terminology Guidebook

## Table of Contents

The terms that follow are divided into the topics shown below. The page number on which the topic begins is given. Within each topic, the terms are arranged alphabetically.

# Introduction / Nutritional Methods

**1. atrophy**

Wasting of tissue.

**2. balance study**

Laboratory study to measure intake and excretion of a nutrient in an organism on a controlled diet.

**3. basic four food groups**

A dietary guideline that specifies daily servings needed from four major food groups.

**4. blind experiment**

Study in which participants do not know whether they are in the experimental or control group.

**5. calorie**

Quantity of heat needed to raise the temperature of one gram water one degree Celsius.

**6. cariogenicity index**

Degree to which a food promotes tooth decay.

**7. control group**

Group of subjects not receiving treatment but as similar as possible to those receiving treatment.

**8. correlation**

Simultaneous change of two variables in the same direction.

**9. diet record**

A method of diet measurement in which the subject writes down kinds and amounts of all foods and drinks consumed.

**10. dietary goals**

Governmental recommendations (in U. S. and Canada) for improving the diet of the public.

**11.  dietary history**

A record of food intake over a period of time.

**12.  dietary recall**

Method for measuring the diet in which the subject is asked to remember their consumption over a given period of time.

**13.  double blind**

Study in which neither participants nor scientists know who is in experimental and who is in control group.

**14.  enriched food**

A food having nutrients added usually to compensate for what has been removed during processing.

**15.  epidemiology**

Study of incidence and distribution of diseases.

**16.  essential nutrient**

Nutrient the body cannot make and must obtain from diet.

**17.  food**

Material ingested that has nutrient value.

**18.  food composition tables**

A list of the average amounts of fat, protein, vitamins, etc. that are contained in given amounts of various foods.

**19.  food disappearance study**

An annual data collection effort that measures the amount of food in the civilian distribution system.

**20.  fortified food**

A food having nutrients added usually in quantities greater than were present naturally.

**21.  health**

A state of complete mental, physical, and social well-being, and not merely the absence of disease.

**22.   health food**

A term with no legal meaning sometimes used to imply that a food has some special health-promoting power.

**23.   health promotion**

Activities that help people to change their behavior and life-style in ways that help them reach maximum health.

**24.   homeostasis**

Maintenance of internal body conditions within a normal tolerable range.

**25.   household consumption study**

Research concerning nutritional behavior in which the data collection efforts actually occur inside people's homes.

**26.   hypertrophy**

An increase in cell size.

**27.   immune system**

The body's system that defends against infectious agents and foreign substances.

**28.   immunity**

The body's ability to defend against infectious agents and foreign substances.

**29.   kilocalorie**

Heat required to raise the temperature of one kilogram of water one degree Celsius.

**30.   lean tissue**

Tissue of the body that is not predominately fat.

**31.   longitudinal study**

Research study in which subjects are observed regularly over a period of time.

**32.   mineral**

Inorganic substance.

### 33. natural food

A term with no legal meaning to describe food having nearly all its original farm-grown properties.

### 34. nutrient

A substance present in or added to a food to improve its dietary value.

### 35. nutrient density

The number and quantity of nutrients in a food relative to other foods.

### 36. nutrition

The act of providing substances needed for good health through food ingestion.

### 37. organic

Containing carbon.

### 38. organic food

A term with no legal meaning to describe food grown without the application of fertilizers or pesticides.

### 39. overnutrition

Intake of too much energy or nutrients.

### 40. placebo

An inert substance given to give comfort to recipient; given to control group in blind study, for example.

### 41. placebo effect

Improvement in condition after receiving a placebo.

### 42. primary deficiency

The lack of a nutrient because of an inadequate diet.

### 43. principle of variety

Eating a wide variety of foods over several days; principle of dilution.

**44. prospective study**

Research study in which subjects are measured initially and after some time to find what changes have occured.

**45. randomization**

Selection of subjects in a way that each is equally likely to enter experimental or control group.

**46. recommended dietary allowance (RDA)**

Daily intake of a nutrient recommended by the National Research Council.

**47. refined food**

A food with coarse parts removed.

**48. replication**

Collecting of the same kind of data while repeating an experiment.

**49. requirement**

In nutrition, the minimum amount of a substance that will prevent specific signs of deficiency.

**50. retrospective study**

Research study in which subjects are measured and their history is used to explain differences among them.

**51. risk factor**

Attribute correlated with a disease, but not necessarily known to cause it.

**52. secondary deficiency**

The lack of a nutrient because of a factor other than inadequate diet.

**53. sign**

An abnormal condition observable in a patient by another person.

**54. staple**

A food consumed almost daily.

**55. subclinical**

A disorder, such as a nutritional deficiency, with no observable effects.

**56. subclinical deficiency**

Inapparent lack of a nutrient.

**57. supplement**

On labels, a nutrient that has been added in an amount greater than 50 percent of the U. S. RDA.

**58. symptom**

An abnormal condition reported by a patient.

**59. syndrome**

An assortment of symptoms that occur together.

**60. synergism**

A situation in which the combined effect of two factors is greater than the sum of their individual effects.

**61. undernutrition**

Intake of too little energy or nutrients.

**62. variable**

Factor that can change in an experiment.

**63. vitamin**

Essential organic nutrient needed in a very small amount.

**64. whole grain**

Unrefined grain or product made from it.

# General Chemistry

**65. acid**

An ionizing substance that donates hydrogen ions.

**66. alkaline**

Basic, able to accept hydrogen ions.

**67. anion**

A negatively charge ion.

**68. atom**

Smallest particle that retains properties of an element.

**69. atomic number**

The number of protons in the nucleus of an atom.

**70. atomic weight**

The total number of protons and neutrons in an atom; the average number if there are isotopes of the element.

**71. base**

An ionizing substance that accepts hydrogen ions or reacts with an acid to form a salt.

**72. bioenergetics**

The science of energy changes in living systems.

**73. buffer**

A substance that resists pH change by holding or releasing hydrogen ions in a solution.

**74. catalyst**

A substance that increases a chemical reaction rate.

**75. cation**

A positively charged ion.

**76. cis-fatty acid**

Fatty acid in which carbon chains extend from same side of the double bond.

**77. colloid**

Glue-like; a particle in a colloidal dispersion.

**78. colloidal dispersion**

A state of matter with small particles suspended in a medium.

**79. compound**

A substance with two or more elements combined in definite proportion.

**80. concentration gradient**

A range of differences in the concentration of a solute.

**81. covalent bond**

A chemical bond formed by shared electrons between two atoms.

**82. dehydration**

Removal of water.

**83. electron**

A negatively charged particle that continually moves around the nucleus of an atom.

**84. element**

A fundamental unit of matter.

**85. enzyme**

A protein that increases the rate of a chemical reaction in a living organism.

86. **fructose**

Monosaccharide found in many fruits and product of breakdown of sucrose (table sugar).

87. **functional group**

A component of a molecule that participates in a chemical reaction.

88. **galactose**

Monosaccharide found in the lactose (milk sugar).

89. **glucose**

Monosaccharide found in blood and product of breakdown of starch and glycogen.

90. **glycoprotein**

A molecule that contains both carbohydrate and protein components.

91. **gram molecular weight**

The quantity of a substance (in grams) equal to its molecular weight.

92. **hydrogen bond**

Weak covalent bond between hydrogen and another element, such as oxygen or nitrogen.

93. **hydrolysis**

The splitting of a molecule with the addition of water.

94. **hydrophilic**

Attacted to water.

95. **hydrophobic**

Tending to avoid water.

96. **hyperosmotic**

Having higher osmotic pressure .

**97. hypertonic**

Causing movement of water out of cells.

**98. hyposmotic**

Having lower osmotic pressure .

**99. hypotonic**

Causing movement of water into cells.

**100. ion**

A charged atom or group of atoms.

**101. ionic bond**

A chemical bond with atoms held together by the attraction of unlike charges.

**102. isomer**

A molecule having the same kinds and number of atoms as another molecule, but arranged differently.

**103. isosmotic**

Having the same osmotic pressure as a reference solution.

**104. isotonic**

Causing no net water movement across a cell membrane.

**105. isotope**

An atom having a different number of neutrons than certain other atoms of the same element.

**106. lactose**

Disaccharide consisting of glucose and galactose; milk sugar.

**107. lactose intolerance**

Inherited inability to digest lactose because of a missing enzyme.

**108. ligand**

That which binds to a receptor.

**109. macromolecule**

A molecule containing thousands of atoms.

**110. maltose**

Disaccharide consisting of two glucose units.

**111. mixture**

Two or more substances combined in any proportions and retaining their individual properties.

**112. mole**

A gram molecular weight.

**113. molecule**

The smallest quantity of a substance that retains its chemical properties.

**114. neutron**

An uncharged particle in the nucleus of an atom.

**115. nonpolar**

Uncharged; lacking polarity.

**116. nucleus**

Central part of an atom or a cell.

**117. osmosis**

Diffusion of water from its own higher to a lower concentration.

**118. osmotic pressure**

Pressure created by osmosis.

### 119. oxidation

Addition of oxygen or loss of electrons in a chemical reaction.

### 120. pH

A scale for expressing acidity or alkalinity; the negative logarithm of the hydrogen ion concentration.

### 121. potential energy

Energy due to position and capable of being released, as in a rock at the top of a hill.

### 122. product

A substance formed, as in a chemical reaction or process.

### 123. proton

A positively charged particle in the nucleus of an atom.

### 124. radiation

Spreading from a center; giving off electromagnetic particles and waves.

### 125. radical

Unstable (usually charged intermediate) in a chemical process.

### 126. reactant

A substance that is changed by a chemical reaction.

### 127. reduction

Gain of an electron or loss of oxygen in a chemical reaction.

### 128. solute

A dissolved substance.

### 129. solution

A liquid containing dissolved substances.

**130. solvent**

A substance in which other substances can dissolve.

**131. specific heat**

The amount of heat needed to increase the temperature of a specific volume of substance one degree Celsius.

**132. sucrose**

Disaccharide consisting of glucose and fructose; table sugar.

**133. surface tension**

Resistance to rupture by the surface film of a liquid.

**134. tonicity**

The degree to which fluid can move into or out of cells.

**135. trans-fatty acid**

Fatty acid in which the carbon chains extend from opposite sides of the double bond.

**136. valence**

An ion's charge.

# Carbohydrates

**137. addiction**

An uncontrollable physiological need for a substance, such as alcohol or other drugs.

**138. amylase**

An enzyme that digests starch.

**139. available carbohydrate**

Carbohydrate that can be digested by human enzymes.

**140. carboholic**

A popular term used to suggest that a person is addicted to carbohydrate, especially sugar; sucroholic.

**141. carbohydrate**

An organic compound having several alcohol groups and an aldehyde or ketone group.

**142. carbohydrate loading**

Procedure used by some athletes to store more than their usual amount of glycogen.

**143. cellulose**

A polymer of glucose made by plant cells and serving as a component of a plant's structure.

**144. complex carbohydrate**

Polysaccharide, such as starch or glycogen.

**145. crude fiber**

Plant fiber remaining after extraction with dilute acid and dilute base.

**146. cytoplasm**

Cell substance, excluding the nucleus.

**147. dextrin**

One of several short chains of glucose units from digestion of starch.

**148. dietary fiber**

Plant fiber remaining after a food is digested by human enzymes.

**149. disaccharide**

A molecule having two sugar (saccharide) units held together by a glycosidic bond.

**150. fiber**

A group of substances found in foods drived from plants that are not digested by human enzymes.

**151. gliadin**

A protein in wheat and some other grains that damages the intestinal mucosa in sensitive individuals.

**152. glucagon**

A hormone that raises blood glucose.

**153. gluten**

A substance containing gliadin found in wheat and some other grains.

**154. glycogen**

A polymer of glucose made by animal cells.

**155. gum**

A carbohydrate-like fiber found in some plant foods.

**156. hemicellulose**

A polysaccharide fiber found in plant foods.

**157. hormone**

A regulatory substance from an endocrine cell that is transported in the blood to its target cells.

## 158. hyperglycemia

Abnormally high blood glucose concentration.

## 159. hypoglycemia

Abnormally low blood glucose concentration.

## 160. hypoglycemic

Pertaining to low blood glucose; an agent that lowers blood glucose.

## 161. insulin

A hormone from the pancreas that causes cells to take in glucose and stimulates protein synthesis.

## 162. insulin shock

Unconsciousness due to an insulin overdose that suddenly lowers blood glucose.

## 163. islet of Langerhans

Cluster of hormone-secreting cells in the pancreas.

## 164. lactase

An enzyme that digests lactose.

## 165. lignin

A carbohydrate-like fiber found in foods from woody plants.

## 166. maltase

Enzyme that digests maltose, a disaccharide from starch.

## 167. monosaccharide

A simple sugar.

## 168. mucilage

A carbohydrate-like fiber found in some plant foods.

**169. pectin**

A polysaccharide fiber found in plant foods.

**170. polydipsia**

Excessive fluid intake.

**171. polymer**

A molecule consisting of repeating units.

**172. polyphagia**

Excessive eating.

**173. polysaccharide**

A molecule consisting of many saccharide units connected by glycosidic bonds.

**174. polyuria**

Excessive urine production.

**175. positive reinforcer**

A reward that increases the likelihood a behavior will be repeated, as occurs in eating of sweets.

**176. postingestive effect**

The effect a food produces after it has been eaten, such as the eating sugar raising the blood glucose level.

**177. seasonal affective disorder (SAD)**

Depression attributed to lessened light in fall and winter.

**178. simple carbohydrate**

Monosaccharide; sugar.

**179. sprue**

Inflammation and partial destruction of the gastrointestinal mucosa.

**180. starch**

A polymer of glucose made by plant cells and serving as a form of energy storage.

**181. stereoisomer**

Compound having the same kind and number of atoms as another compound, but in a different spatial arrangement.

**182. sucrase**

An enzyme that digests sucrose.

**183. unavailable carbohydrate**

Carbohydrate that cannot be digested by human enzymes.

# Lipids

**184. acetylcholine**

A substance derived from choline that transmits signals between neurons and from neurons to muscle cells.

**185. aldosterone**

An adrenocortical hormone that increases reabsorption of sodium.

**186. anabolic steroid**

A synthetic hormone that increases muscle size.

**187. androgen**

A molecule with male hormone activity.

**188. arachidonic acid**

A twenty-carbon polyunsaturated fatty acid.

**189. atherosclerosis**

Obstruction of arteries by hardened plaque deposits.

**190. cholesterol**

Sterol found in meat, dairy products, and eggs.

**191. cholesteryl esterase**

Enzyme that breaks ester bonds between a fatty acid and cholesterol.

**192. chylomicron**

A particle made of lipids and protein in the intestinal mucosa and released into lacteals.

**193. corticosterone**

A steroid hormone from adrenal cortex.

### 194. cortisol

An adrenocortical hormone that helps regulate carbohydrate metabolism and counteracts inflammation.

### 195. emulsification

Process by which bile salts cause fat droplets from foods to break into smaller particles.

### 196. emulsify

To disperse and stabilize fat in a liquid solution.

### 197. enterohepatic circulation

Return of bile salts to the liver and their resecretion in bile.

### 198. epinephrine

Main hormone from the adrenal medulla.

### 199. essential fatty acid

Fatty acid required in the diet because the body cannot make it.

### 200. estrogen

One of several active molecules that stimulate development of female organs and secondary sexual characteristics.

### 201. fat

Triglyceride mixture.

### 202. fatty acid

A long hydrocarbon chain with a carboxyl group at one end.

### 203. glycolipid

A molecule that contains both carbohydrate and lipid components.

### 204. high density lipoprotein (HDL)

Lipoprotein that seems to carry cholesterol back to the liver, it is also known as alpha-lipoprotein.

**205. hormone sensitive lipase**

Enzyme inside adipose cells that releases fatty acids when nutrients in blood decrease.

**206. hydrogenation**

The creation of a saturated fat by the addition of hydrogen atoms.

**207. lecithin**

A phospholipid characteristic of animal tissues.

**208. lipase**

An enzyme that breaks down lipids.

**209. lipid**

Fat or fatlike substance.

**210. lipophilic**

Soluble in fat; literally, lipid-loving.

**211. lipophobic**

Lipid-fearing.

**212. lipoprotein**

A molecule made of lipid and protein.

**213. lipoprotein lipase**

Enzyme on the surface of some cells that hydrolyzes triglycerides passing by in the bloodstream.

**214. low density lipoprotein (LDL)**

Substance that transports cholesterol from cells in the liver to other cells.

**215. micelle**

A small fat droplet in chyme.

**216. mixed triglyceride**

A triglyceride containing more than one type of fatty acid.

**217. monounsaturated fatty acid**

Fatty acid that has one double bond between carbons and lacks two hydrogen atoms.

**218. myelin**

An insulating substance deposited around axons.

**219. oleic acid**

An 18-carbon fatty acid having one point of unsaturation.

**220. omega-3 fatty acid**

A type of fat found in fish that has been linked with lower blood pressure, reduced clotting, and lower cholesterol.

**221. omega-6 fatty acid**

A fatty acid in which the first double bond is six carbons away from its methyl end.

**222. phospholipid**

A lipid made of glycerol, fatty acids, and phosphoric acid.

**223. plaque**

A sheetlike deposit.

**224. polar compound**

A molecule having a charged area or polarity.

**225. polyunsaturated fat**

Fat that is made up of triglycerides containing a high percentage of PUFAs.

**226. polyunsaturated fatty acid (PUFA)**

A fatty acid that has two or more double bonds between carbons and lacks four or more hydrogen atoms.

**227. progesterone**

A hormone that helps to maintain pregnancy.

**228. prostaglandin**

A substance derived from the fatty acid arachidonic acid that acts over short distances as a chemical messenger.

**229. saturated fatty acid**

A fatty acid lacking double bonds in the carbon chain and being saturated with hydrogen.

**230. saturation**

Condition of having all chemical affinities satisfied.

**231. steroid**

A sterol with certain modifications.

**232. sterol**

A type of complex lipid having a four-ring structure.

**233. taurine**

An amino acid derivative that conjugates with bile acids.

**234. testosterone**

A male hormone.

**235. thromboxane**

A prostaglandin made from arachidonic acid and that promotes blood clotting.

**236. triacylglycerol**

A lipid molecule containing glycerol and three fatty acids.

**237. triglyceride**

A common name for a triacylglycerol.

## 238. unsaturated fatty acid

Fatty acid with pairs of hydrogen atoms replaced by double bonds in the carbon chain.

## 239. very low density lipoproteins (VLDL)

Lipoproteins that transport triglycerides to body tissues.

# Proteins

**240. actin**

A contractile protein.

**241. adrenalin**

A hormone secreted by the adrenal glands.

**242. adrenocorticotropic hormone**

A hormone that stimulates the adrenal cortex to secrete hormones.

**243. albumin**

A small protein made in the liver and released into blood.

**244. allergen**

A substance capable of eliciting an allergic reaction.

**245. amino acid**

A molecule having both acid and amino functional groups.

**246. aminopeptidase**

An enzyme that digests peptides from the amino end.

**247. antibodies**

Proteins that attack foreign matter within the body.

**248. biological value**

Measure of the degree to which amino acids are incorporated into new protein within the body.

**249. calmodulin**

An intracellular calcium carrier molecule.

**250. carboxypeptidase**

A proteolytic enzyme that digests peptides from the carboxyl end.

**251. chemical score (of a protein)**

A quality rating based on a comparison of a protein's amino acid pattern with that of a reference protein.

**252. cholinesterase**

An enzyme that degrades acetylcholine.

**253. chymotrypsin**

A proteolytic enzyme from the pancreas.

**254. collagen**

A fibrous protein in connective tissue.

**255. complementary proteins**

Proteins in which the amino acids missing from one are supplied by the other.

**256. complete protein**

A protein that contains adequate amounts of all the amino acids people need.

**257. denaturation**

An alteration in the shape and properties of a protein molecule.

**258. deoxyribonucleic acid (DNA)**

A nucleic acid in chromosomes that directs protein synthesis and transmits genetic information to a new generation.

**259. digestibility (of protein)**

The degree to which amino acids are available for absorption from breakdown of a protein.

**260. dipeptidase**

An enzyme that digests dipeptides to amino acids.

## 261. dipeptide

A molecule of two amino acids held together by a peptide bond.

## 262. endogenous nitrogen

Nitrogen that enters the body from the environment.

## 263. endogenous protein

Protein that has been broken down and is traveling through the body.

## 264. endorphin

A peptide that binds to opiate receptors in the brain.

## 265. enkephalin

A peptide derived from endorphin that binds to opiate receptors in the brain.

## 266. enterokinase

A proteolytic enzyme from the intestinal mucosa.

## 267. essential amino acid

Amino acid required in the diet because the body cannot make it.

## 268. exogenous nitrogen

Nitrogen from food; nitrogen from outside of the body.

## 269. fibrin

A fibrous protein that forms a network in a blood clot.

## 270. fibrinogen

Inactive fibrin.

## 271. fruitarian

Strict vegetarian who eats mainly fruits.

### 272. globin

A globular protein found in hemoglobin and certain other biological molecules.

### 273. globulin

A globular protein, including many in the plasma.

### 274. glycine

An amino acid with the simplest chemical structure.

### 275. gruel

A usually thin cooked cereal made by boiling meal.

### 276. high-quality protein

Complete and easily-digestible protein having amino acids in proportions that people need.

### 277. histamine

A derivative of the amino acid histidine released by injured cells that causes vasodilation and bronchial constriction.

### 278. kwashiorkor

Protein deficiency, usually in young children.

### 279. lacto-ovo-vegetarian

A vegetarian who eats products from living animals, such as eggs, milk, and cheese.

### 280. limiting amino acid

The amino acid that is in shortest supply relative to the other amino acids needed for protein synthesis.

### 281. macrobiotic diet

A diet consisting mainly of whole grain and vegetable products thought by some to increase spritual enlightment.

### 282. meat replacement

A vegetable protein product made to look and taste like meat.

**283. melanin**

A dark brown pigment of hair and skin.

**284. metabolic nitrogen**

Nitrogen in molecules from the body's metabolic processes.

**285. mucin**

A glycoprotein in ground substance and mucous secretions.

**286. mucous**

Pertaining to mucus.

**287. mutual supplementation**

The combining of two protein-containing foods in a meal so that together they supply all essential amino acids.

**288. myoglobin**

A pigmented protein that binds oxygen in muscle tissue.

**289. myosin**

A protein that comprises thick filaments of a myofibril.

**290. net protein utilization**

Proportion of protein eaten that is actually used by cells.

**291. neurotransmitter**

A chemical substance from one neuron that transmits a signal to another neuron at a synapse.

**292. nitrogen balance study**

A procedure for measurement of the body's protein usage.

**293. nonessential amino acids**

The thirteen amino acids that can be made by the human body when essential ones are provided in the diet.

**294. nutritional yeast**

A fortified food containing protein, B vitamins, and iron used to increase quality of a vegetarian diet.

**295. oligopeptide**

A string of between four and ten amino acids.

**296. opsin**

A protein that combines with retinine in the retina.

**297. peptide bond**

A chemical bond between the amino group of one amino acid and the carboxyl group of another.

**298. permease**

An enzyme that assists in the transport of a substance into a cell.

**299. polypeptide**

A chain of amino acids held together by peptide bonds.

**300. procarboxypeptidase**

Inactive carboxypeptidase.

**301. prolactin**

A hormone that stimulates milk secretion.

**302. protease**

A protein-digesting enzyme that is secreted into the small intestine.

**303. protein**

A polymer of amino acids.

**304. protein efficiency ratio**

A measure of how well a particular protein supports growth.

### 305. protein turnover

The breakdown and resynthesis of a protein molecule.

### 306. protein-calorie malnutrition

Disease caused by a deficiency of protein and calories.

### 307. protein-energy malnutrition

Impairment due to lack of both protein and energy-yielding foods in the diet.

### 308. prothrombin

A blood protein converted to thrombin in the presence of calcium ions.

### 309. reference protein

Egg protein used as a standard for measuring the quality of other proteins.

### 310. retinene

A carotenoid pigment that binds to opsin.

### 311. rhodopsin

A light-sensitive protein found in rods of the retina.

### 312. secretagogue

Substance that stimulates secretion of digestive juices.

### 313. specificity

The attribute of being specific.

### 314. thrombin

An enzyme that activates fibrinogen to fibrin in the blood clotting mechanism.

### 315. thromboplastin

A substance released from injured tissue that participates in blood clotting.

### 316. transferase

Any of the enzymes that catalyze the transfer of an organic group from one compound to another.

### 317. tripeptide

Three amino acids bonded by peptide bonds.

### 318. trypsin

A proteolytic enzyme released from the pancreas.

### 319. trypsinogen

Inactive trypsin.

### 320. tryptophan

Essential amino acid that is a precursor for serotonin.

### 321. vegan

A vegetarian who eats only foods derived from plant sources.

# Vitamins

**322. acid phosphatase**

Enzyme that degrades calcium phosphate and fosters bone degradation.

**323. active site**

Surface region of an enzyme where its substrate attaches.

**324. alkaline phosphatase**

Enzyme that synthesizes calcium phosphate and fosters bone deposition.

**325. anemia**

Lack of hemoglobin that reduces the oxygen carrying capacity of the blood.

**326. antagonist**

An agent that interferes with the action of a substance, such as a drug that antagonizes a vitamin.

**327. antiscorbutic factor**

Original name for vitamin C because of the vitamin's ability to prevent scurvy.

**328. apoenzyme**

A portion of an enzyme without its prosthetic group.

**329. ariboflavinosis**

Riboflavin deficiency.

**330. ascorbic**

Without scurvy.

**331. avidin**

Protein in eggwhites that binds biotin.

**332. beriberi**

Thiamine deficiency.

**333. beta-carotene**

A precursor of vitamin A found in plants.

**334. bilirubin**

A bile pigment derived from the breakdown of hemoglobin.

**335. biotin**

Vitamin required for fat synthesis.

**336. bone meal**

Powered bone sometimes used to supply calcium.

**337. carotene**

Yellow substance that usually has vitamin A activity.

**338. carpal tunnel sydrome**

Pain and numbness in the hand due to pressure on a nerve and maybe associated with vitamin B6 deficiency.

**339. cheliosis**

Inflammation around nose and lips, cracking of corners of mouth.

**340. Chinese restaurant syndrome**

Intolerance to the food additive monosodium glutamate, possibly associated with vitamin B6 deficiency.

**341. chlorophyll**

Green pigment in plants which transfers light energy to molecules used in photosynthesis.

**342. coenzyme**

A molecule that works with an enzyme and is required for the enzyme to function.

**343. cones**

Retinal cells that respond to bright light and are responsible for color vision.

**344. cornea**

Transparent membrane that covers the outside of the front of the eye.

**345. cruciferous vegetable**

A plant with cross-shaped blossoms in which edible parts protect against cancer in laboratory animals.

**346. dentin**

Relatively soft material underlying tooth enamel.

**347. dessicated liver**

Powdered form of liver tissue sold in health food stores having no proven value.

**348. enamel**

Hard coating on the outside of a tooth.

**349. epithelial cell**

Cell in a tissue that covers a surface or lines an organ.

**350. epithelium**

A thin tissue that lines hollow organs or covers surfaces.

**351. ergocalciferol**

A kind of vitamin D found in plants.

**352. erythocyte**

Red blood cell.

**353. fat-soluble vitamins**

Vitamins A, D, E and K.

### 354. fibrocystic breast disease

Presence of harmless painful lumps of fibrous tissue in breasts, which may respond to vitamin E.

### 355. folacin

Vitamin needed to help transfer single carbon groups.

### 356. follicle

Cup-like group of cells, such as that from which a hair grows.

### 357. follicular hyperkeratosis

Deposition of keratin around hair follicles.

### 358. fontanel

Open space between bones in a baby's skull before the bones have grown together.

### 359. food fortification

The addition of vitamins or minerals to food products.

### 360. food supplements

Vitamins and minerals that may be added to the diet, often in pill or capsule form.

### 361. glossitis

Swelling and cracking of tongue.

### 362. gout

Metabolic disorder involving precipitation of uric acid crystals in joints and other tissues.

### 363. granola

A cereal consisting of a mixture of whole grains.

### 364. hemolysis

Break down of erythrocytes (red blood cells).

### 365. hemophilia

Hereditary impairment of blood clotting due to body's inability to make one or more blood clotting factors.

### 366. hemorrhagic disease

Impaired blood clotting due to vitamin K deficiency.

### 367. holoenzyme

A functional enzyme complete with its prosthetic group.

### 368. hyperbilirubinemia

Jaundice.

### 369. hypercalcemia

Excessive blood calcium that can be caused by very high doses of vitamin D.

### 370. hyperkeratinization

Excess deposition of keratin in epithelial cells.

### 371. hypervitaminosis A

Toxic effects of excess vitamin A.

### 372. hypervitaminosis D

Toxic effects of excess vitamin D.

### 373. intermittent claudication

Nocturnal leg cramps and pain while walking, which may respond to vitamin E.

### 374. international unit

Vitamin A activity as the effect of giving a known amount of a substance to a vitamin A deprived animal.

### 375. intrinsic factor (IF)

Substance produced by the gastric mucosa that is necessary for the transport and absorption of vitamin B12.

**376. jaundice**

Yellowing of the skin that is a symptom of liver disease.

**377. kelp**

A seaweed commonly used in food in Japan.

**378. keratin**

A durable protein substance found in hair and nails.

**379. keratomalacia**

Blindness due to damage to the cornea.

**380. kernicterus**

Damage to brain tissue from accumulation of bile pigments.

**381. lysosome**

A sac of degradative enzymes.

**382. megadose**

Excessively large dose of some substance, vitamin C, for example.

**383. menadione**

A synthetic, quick acting form of vitamin K.

**384. mineralization**

Process by which minerals such as calcium and phosphorus crystallize and are deposited in the matrix of bones.

**385. mucopolysaccharide**

A molecule containing many sugar units and amine groups.

**386. mucosa**

Membranes that line the surfaces of body tissues.

**387. mucus**

Substance secreted by the epithelial cells of the mucosa.

**388. niacin**

B vitamin used to synthesize the coenzyme NAD.

**389. niacin equivalent**

Amount of niacin in food including niacin capable of being made from tryptophan in the food.

**390. night blindness**

A condition in which vision is impaired in dimly lit places, often caused by a lack of vitamin A.

**391. nutritional muscular dystrophy**

A kind of muscle atrophy seen in some animals (but not in humans) during vitamin E deprivation.

**392. osteoblast**

A cell that builds bone.

**393. osteoclast**

A cell that destroys bone during its growth.

**394. osteomalacia**

Adult bone softening as a result of a vitamin deficiency.

**395. oxidant**

Molecule (including oxygen itself) that oxidizes other molecules.

**396. pantothenic acid**

B vitamin used to synthesize coenzyme A.

**397. pellagra**

Niacin deficiency.

**398. pernicious anemia**

Anemia due to a lack of intrinsic factor and therefore vitamin B12.

**399. peroxidation**

Making of hydrogen peroxide and other molecules with large quantities of oxygen.

**400. pharmacological effect**

Effect of a vitamin or other agent present in a very large amount and having an effect like a drug.

**401. photon**

A unit of light energy.

**402. photosynthesis**

Manufacture of carbohydrates in plants from carbon dioxide and water and light energy.

**403. physiological effect**

Effect of a vitamin or other nutrient present in a normal amount.

**404. pigeon breast**

Abnormal rib cage shape seen in children with rickets.

**405. promoter**

An agent that fosters development of cancer initiated by another agent.

**406. prosthetic group**

A functional component (such as a coenzyme) physically attached to an enzyme.

**407. provitamin**

A molecule that can be converted into an active vitamin.

**408. rachitic rosary**

Beadlike structure on the ribs of children with rickets.

**409. rebound scurvy**

Development of scurvy when large doses of vitamin C are terminated.

**410. retina**

Layer of cells at the back of the inside of the eye, consisting of rods and cones.

**411. retinol (retinal)**

An active form of vitamin A.

**412. retinol equivalent**

Vitamin A activity as the amount of retinol a substance with vitamin A activity will yield after conversion in body.

**413. riboflavin**

Heat-labile B vitamin used to synthesize the coenzyme FAD.

**414. rod**

Retinal cell that responds to dim light and conveys blank and white images.

**415. spirulina**

An edible product made from blue-green algae.

**416. thiamine**

A water-soluble B vitamin used to synthesize cocarboxylase.

**417. tocopherol**

A type of alcohol, of which vitamin E is an example.

**418. vitamin A**

Vitamin needed to synthesize visual pigments and maintain epithelial cells.

**419. vitamin B12**

Vitamin that helps form genetic material and red blood cells and helps in nervous system function; cyanocobalamin.

**420. vitamin B6**

Group of related molecules--pyridoxine, pyridoxal, and pyridoxamine) required for action of many kinds of enzymes.

**421. vitamin C**

A vitamin that is important in forming collagen and is found in citrus fruits and dark green vegetables; ascorbic acid.

**422. vitamin D**

A vitamin that facilitates calcium absorption.

**423. vitamin D3**

A natural substance formed by the action of sunlight on a cholesterol derivative in the skin; cholecalciferol.

**424. vitamin E**

Vitamin that acts as an antioxidant.

**425. vitamin K**

Vitamin needed for synthesis of some blood clotting factors.

**426. vitamin-D-resistant rickets**

Deficient bone mineralization due to lack of absorption of vitamin D.

**427. Wernicke-Korsokoff syndrome**

Condition that sometimes develops in alcoholics, involving a greater need for thiamine combined with lower intake.

**428. wheat germ**

Highly nutritious portion of a wheat grain from which a new plant arises.

**429. withdrawal reaction**

Effect of no longer receiving a substance such as a drug or large amounts of a vitamin formerly received.

**430. xerophthalmia**

Dry eye, such as results from vitamin A deficiency.

## 431. xerosis

Drying of the cornea.

# Minerals and Water

**432. acid-base balance**

Maintenance of body fluid pH withing a normal range.

**433. acidophilus milk**

Milk to which the bacterium Lactobacillus acidophilus has been added.

**434. acidosis**

Condition due to low blood pH.

**435. alkalosis**

Condition due to high blood pH.

**436. antidiuretic hormone (ADH)**

Substance secreted by the pituitary that makes the kidney conserve water.

**437. apoferritin**

A protein that carries iron.

**438. biliverdin**

A green bile pigment from hemoglobin breakdown.

**439. binders**

Substances found in foods that combine with minerals and some other nutrients to form nonabsorbable complexes.

**440. blood transferrin**

A carrier protein that transports iron in the blood.

**441. calciferol**

Steroid having vitamin D activity.

### 442. calcitonin

A hormone that lowers blood calcium.

### 443. calcium rigor

Muscle stiffness due to elevated blood calcium.

### 444. calcium tetany

Intermittent muscle spasms due to depleted blood calcium.

### 445. chloride

Chlorine in ionic form.

### 446. contamination iron

Iron in the diet from cooking pans and soils.

### 447. contraction alkalosis

Abnormal increase in the blood pH caused by a decrease in body fluid volume.

### 448. cretinism

Congenital deficiency of thyroid hormone.

### 449. cytochrome

An enzyme that transports electrons in reduced iron ions.

### 450. diastole

Relaxation of heart chambers during which they fill with blood.

### 451. diuretic

A drug that stimulates the kidneys to excrete more water; popularly called a water pill.

### 452. electrolyte

Substance that ionizes and conducts electricity.

**453. erythrocyte**

Red blood cell.

**454. erythrocyte protoporphyrin**

A precursor molecule in hemoglobin synthesis.

**455. extracellular**

Outside a cell.

**456. ferric ion**

An iron ion with 3 positive charges; oxidized iron.

**457. ferritin**

A molecule made up of the protein apoferritin and iron.

**458. ferrous ion**

An iron ion with 2 positive charged; reduced iron.

**459. fluid regulation**

Maintenance of body fluid volumes within normal ranges.

**460. fluorapatite**

Bone mineral in which fluoride has replaced some hydroxy groups.

**461. fluorosis**

Mottling of teeth due to excess fluoride present during tooth development.

**462. galvanizing**

The coating of metal with zinc to prevent rust.

**463. gastroferrin**

An iron-binding protein that transports iron from the stomach lumen to mucosal cells.

**464. geophagia**

The practice of eating clay.

**465. glucose tolerance factor (GTF)**

A chromium containing substance which seems to counteract impaired glucose metabolism in some older patients.

**466. goiter**

Enlarged thyroid gland.

**467. goitrogen**

A substance that antagonizes thyroid hormone.

**468. hard water**

Water containing many calcium and magnesium ions.

**469. hematocrit**

A measure of the volume of erythrocytes in a sample of whole blood.

**470. heme**

An iron-containing pigment in hemoglobin that binds oxygen.

**471. hemoglobin**

An iron-containing protein in erythrocytes that binds oxygen.

**472. hemosiderin**

A molecule that binds and stores iron.

**473. hydroxyapatite**

Major crystalline form of calcium and phosphorus found in bone.

**474. hypertension**

High blood pressure.

### 475. hypochromic

Having too little color.

### 476. insensible

Imperceptible.

### 477. intracellular

Inside a cell.

### 478. iron overload

Toxic effects of an excess of iron in the tissues.

### 479. Keshan disease

Condition related to a deficiency of selenium.

### 480. leukocyte ferritin

Quantity of ferritin (and potential iron binding) in leukocytes.

### 481. major mineral

Any mineral that is needed in an amount greater than one hundred miligrams per day.

### 482. meat-fish-poultry (MFP) factor

A substance found in meat, fish, and poultry that fosters iron absorption.

### 483. metabolic acidosis

A lowering of blood pH because of a metabolic disorder.

### 484. metabolic alkalosis

A raising of blood pH because of a metabolic disorder.

### 485. metalloenzyme

An enzyme that contains one or more metal ions

### 486. metallothionine

A sulfur rich protein that binds zinc.

### 487. microcytic

Having small cells.

### 488. milliequivalent (mEq)

A quantity of a substance having the same number of charges **as 1 mg of hydrogen.**

### 489. minor mineral

Any trace element needed in an amount no greater than a few milligrams per day.

### 490. molybdenum

A trace element that forms part of certain metalloenzymes.

### 491. mucosal ferritin

A protein that binds iron in mucosal cells.

### 492. mucosal transferrin

A carrier protein that moves iron across mucosal cells to blood.

### 493. nephron

A functional and structural unit of the kidney.

### 494. obligatory water excretion

Minimum quantity of water the body must excrete daily (about one pint).

### 495. osmoreceptor

Receptor that senses changes in osmolarity.

### 496. ossification

Mineral deposition in the process of bone formation.

**497. osteoporosis**

Abnormal porousness of bone, which makes it fracture-prone.

**498. oxyhemoglobin**

Hemoglobin to which oxygen is bound.

**499. pagophagia**

The practice of eating large quantities of ice.

**500. parathormone**

A hormone from the parathyorid gland that decreases blood calcium.

**501. parathyroid glands**

Glands imbedded in the thyorid gland.

**502. plasma**

The fluid part of blood including inactive clotting factors.

**503. renin**

A kidney secretion that activates angiotensinogen to angiotensin I.

**504. respiratory acidosis**

A lowering of blood pH because of a respiratory disorder.

**505. respiratory alkalosis**

A raising of blood pH because of a respiratory disorder.

**506. rickets**

A failure of bones to harden in childhood because of a calcium deficiency.

**507. salt**

Molecule consisting of positive and negative ions.

**508. scurvy**

A disease due to a vitamin C deficiency.

**509. selectively permeable**

Permitting passage of some substances and not others.

**510. selenium**

A trace element that forms an essential part of certain enzymes.

**511. selenosis**

A disorder caused by toxic levels of selenium in the body.

**512. simple goiter**

Enlarged thyroid gland due to iodine deficiency.

**513. sodium-potassium pump**

Mechanism that actively moves Na ions out of cells and K ions into them against gradients.

**514. soft water**

Water in which calcium and magnesium ions have been replaced by twice as many sodium ions.

**515. systole**

Rhytmical contraction of the heart during which blood is forced onward.

**516. thirst**

The desire to drink.

**517. thirst center**

Hypothalamic nucleus that responds to changes in the blood osmotic pressure, causing drinking behavior.

**518. total iron binding capacity (TIBC)**

Quantity of iron blood can hold based on available transferrin.

### 519. toxic goiter

Enlarged thyroid gland due to a goitrogen.

### 520. trace element

A chemical element normally present in very small amounts in the body.

### 521. transferrin

An iron-transport protein in plasma.

### 522. transferrin saturation

Condition in which transferrin carries as much iron as it can.

### 523. water balance

Quantity of water entering the body should equal the quantity of water leaving the body.

### 524. water intoxication

Presence of too much water in the body.

### 525. Wilson's disease

Adverse inherited condition in which copper accumulates in tissues, causing toxicity.

### 526. zinc-binding ligand

A substance that fosters absorption of zinc.

# Digestion / Absorption / Transport

**527. absorption**

Movement of substances across a membrane.

**528. absorptive**

Concerning absorption.

**529. active transport**

Transport of a substance against a gradient using a carrier molecule, enzyme, and cellular energy.

**530. aneurysm**

The ballooning out of a weakened wall of an artery.

**531. angina**

Pain caused by a reduction in the blood supply to heart muscle.

**532. anus**

An opening through which wastes exit the digestive tract.

**533. aorta**

Large artery that carries blood from the heart to all parts of the body except respiratory structures of lungs.

**534. artery**

A vessel carrying blood away from the heart.

**535. ascites**

Edema in the abdomen.

**536. bicarbonate**

Negatively charged ion that can neutralize hydrogen ions in acidosis.

**537. bile**

Liver secretion that aids in digestion by emulsifying fats.

**538. binding site**

A site where a particular molecule binds to a membrane or other structure.

**539. blood**

Fluid pumped by the heart through a closed system of vessels.

**540. blood-brain barrier**

A specialized capillary structure that limits movement of substances from blood into brain tissue.

**541. bolus**

A mass.

**542. capillaries**

Small vessels connecting arteries to veins.

**543. cardiovascular disease**

A general term for all diseases affecting the heart and blood vessels.

**544. carrier**

A transfer molecule.

**545. carrier saturation**

A condition with all carrier molecules carrying a substance.

**546. cecum**

Blind pouch.

**547. cerebral thrombosis**

Closing of a blood vessel in the brain by a blood clot.

**548. cerebrovascular accident**

A stroke.

**549. chenodeoxycholic acid**

A bile acid.

**550. chief cell**

A gastric gland cell that secretes pepsin into the stomach.

**551. cholecystokinin (CCK)**

Hormone involved in digestion by releasing bile from the gall bladder and enzymes from the pancreas.

**552. cholesystectomy**

Surgical removal of the gallbladder.

**553. cholic acid**

A bile acid.

**554. chyme**

Semiliquid, partially digested food leaving the stomach.

**555. cirrhosis**

Condition in which liver tissue is hardened, orange, and has many dead cells, often from excessive alcohol use.

**556. co-transport**

Movement of two substances across a membrane by the same carrier.

**557. colipase**

An enzyme that assists a lipase.

**558. colitis**

Inflammation of the colon.

**559. colon**

Large intestine from the cecum to the rectum.

**560. constipation**

Difficult and infrequent defecation.

**561. coronary heart disease**

Atherosclerosis in arteries of the heart muscle itself.

**562. coronary thrombosis**

Closing of a blood vessel in heart muscle by a blood clot.

**563. deciduous teeth**

Nonpermanent teeth; 'baby teeth'.

**564. defecation**

Passage of wastes from the rectum outside the body.

**565. deglutition**

Swallowing.

**566. diarrhea**

Excessively frequent, fluid bowel movements.

**567. digestion**

Breakdown of large molecules into smaller ones.

**568. diverticulitis**

Inflamed or infected pouches in the intestinal wall.

**569. diverticulosis**

Presence of pouches in the intestinal wall.

**570. duodenal**

Of the duodenum.

**571. duodenum**

A short part of the small intestine adjacent to stomach that receives secretions from the liver and pancreas.

**572. dysentery**

A gastrointestinal infection characterized by severe diarrhea.

**573. edema**

Swelling of tissues caused by water accumulation outside of blood vessels.

**574. embolus**

Blood clot that has broken loose and traveled to smaller arterial vessels.

**575. endocrine glands**

Glands that secrete their materials into the blood.

**576. endogenous opiate**

Naturally produced substance resembling morphine that exerts a calming effect on the body.

**577. enterogastric reflex**

Neural signal elicited by excessively acidic or fatty chyme that slows stomach peristalsis.

**578. enterogastrone**

Hormone thought to be produced by the intestine to slow peristalsis when fat is present.

**579. epiglottis**

Elastic cartilage that closes the glottis.

**580. esophageal**

Of the esophagus.

**581. esophagus**

Muscular tube between the pharynx and stomach.

**582. facilitated diffusion**

Diffusion down a gradient on a carrier molecule but not requiring cellular energy.

**583. feces**

Digestive waste expelled from the rectum through the anus.

**584. feedback system**

A self-controlling system whereby input produces output that affects the input source, forming a loop.

**585. filtration**

Passage of a fluid across a membrane by mechanical pressure.

**586. gallbladder**

A sac on the underside of the liver where bile is stored.

**587. gallstone**

Deposit of insoluble particles in gallbladder.

**588. gastric**

Of the stomach.

**589. gastric glands**

Exocrine glands in the wall of the stomach that secrete gastric juice.

**590. gastric juice**

Secretion, from exocrine glands into the stomach, that contains three main enzymes: rennin, pepsin and lipase.

**591. gastrin**

A hormone from the stomach lining that circulates in the blood and stimulates HCl secretion.

**592. gastritis**

Stomach inflammation.

**593. gastroesophageal**

Of the stomach and esophagus.

**594. gastrointestinal tract**

Also known as the alimentary canal, it contains the stomach and the intestines.

**595. general adaptation syndrome**

The pattern of responses of the body to stress.

**596. gingiva**

Gums.

**597. gland**

Cell or group of cells that secrete materials for a particular purposes in the body.

**598. haustra**

A saclike protrusion of the wall of the large intestine.

**599. haustral churning**

Motility that pushes the contents of the large intestine from one haustrum to the next.

**600. hepatic**

Of the liver.

**601. hepatic vein**

Vein that returns blood from the liver capilleries to the heart.

**602. hepatitis**

Inflammation of the liver, which can be due to infection or toxic substances.

**603. hernia**

Separation in a muscle layer; rupture.

**604. hiatal**

Related to a gap or fissure.

**605. hydrolase**

An enzyme that catalyzes hydrolysis.

**606. hypoxia**

Oxygen deficiency in cells.

**607. ileostomy**

Surgical opening from the ileum outside the body.

**608. ileum**

Lower part of the small intestine.

**609. infarct**

Blockage of blood flow (usually relates to a tissue).

**610. intestinal**

Of the intestine.

**611. intestinal flora**

Bacteria living in the digestive tract.

**612. intravenous**

Into a vein.

**613. ischemia**

Tissue damage caused by reduced blood flow that leads to lack of oxygen and nutrients and accumulation of wastes.

**614. ischemic heart disease**

Heart disease caused by reduced blood flow to the heart muscle.

**615. jejunum**

Middle part of the small intestine.

**616. lacteal**

Lymph vessel in a villus of the small intestine.

**617. lamina propria**

Connective tissue beneath mucosal epithelium of the intestine.

**618. latent**

Hidden.

**619. lesion**

A localized, abnormal structural change within the body.

**620. lethal**

Deadly.

**621. lingual**

Of the tongue.

**622. liver**

A glandular organ in the upper right side of the abdominal cavity that secretes bile and performs other functions.

**623. lymph**

Body fluid in spaces between cells and outside the vascular system.

**624. lymphatic system**

Loosely organized system carrying fluid that has escaped the vascular system and producing immune responses.

**625. mesentery**

A double membrane continuous with the peritoneum that suspends an abdominal organ.

**626. microvillus**

A cytoplasmic projection of surface membrane of intestinal epithelial cells.

**627. motility**

Ability to move.

**628. multifactorial**

Having many contributing factors.

**629. muscularis**

A layer of muscle in an organ wall; the muscular part of the intestinal mucosa.

**630. myenteric**

Of the muscle layer of the intestine.

**631. myocardial infarction**

Heart muscle damage due to impaired blood flow; a heart attack.

**632. obstruction**

A blocking or clogging.

**633. occlusion**

Blockage of blood flow (usually relates to a blood vessel).

**634. oral**

Of the mouth.

**635. overt**

Out in open.

**636. palatability**

Having a pleasant taste.

**637. pancreas**

A digestive gland that secretes enzymes and hormones.

**638. pancreatic**

Of the pancreas.

**639. pancreatic juice**

Exocrine secretion of the pancreas.

**640. pancreatitis**

Inflammation of the pancreas.

**641. parotid gland**

A large salivary gland inferior to the ear.

**642. passive transport**

A process that moves substances without energy expenditure by the organism.

**643. pepsin**

An enzyme that starts breakdown of protein in the stomach.

**644. peptic ulcer**

A type of lesion in the stomach or duodenum.

**645. periodontal**

Around a tooth.

**646. peristalsis**

Wavelike, propelling contractions along tubular passageways.

## 647. phytate (phytic acid)

Nonnutrient components of seeds that binds with some ions to form insoluble complexes in the intestine.

## 648. plicae circularis

Transverse folding of the mucosa of the small intestine.

## 649. portal triad

A set of three vessels.

## 650. portal vein

Vein that transports blood from the mesentary to capillaries in the liver.

## 651. pyloric

Of the pylorus.

## 652. pylorus

Stomach region attached to the small intestine.

## 653. receptor

A molecular site with which a specific substance can bind.

## 654. rectum

Terminal portion of the digestive tract between the colon and the anal canal.

## 655. rennin

An enzyme in the stomach of calves that digests milk protein.

## 656. ruga

Ridge or fold.

## 657. saline

Salty; a salt solution.

**658. saliva**

Secretion that moistens food in the mouth.

**659. satiety**

A sensation of fullness that causes a person to stop eating.

**660. secretin**

A hormone from the intestinal mucosa that stimulates secretion of bile and pancreatic fluid.

**661. segmentation**

Splitting into segments; contraction of alternate intestinal segments.

**662. sequester**

To take out of circulation, as when proteins bind hydrogen ions.

**663. serosa**

A membranous lining of body cavities that secretes a watery lubricant.

**664. serotonin**

A substance derived from tryptophan that transmits signals between certain neurons, especially in the brain.

**665. sigmoid**

Like the Greek letter sigma.

**666. sphincter**

A ringlike muscle by which a natural orifice opens and closes.

**667. stress**

A threat or perceived threat to one's well-being, which causes a predictable physiological response.

**668. sublingual**

Beneath the tongue.

**669. submucosa**

A layer beneath the intestinal mucosa.

**670. synapse**

A space between neurons across which signals are relayed by neurotransmitters.

**671. taenia coli**

Muscle strip in the colon.

**672. thoracic duct**

Channel through which lymph is conveyed toward the heart.

**673. thrombus**

Blood clot that forms on top of plaque or on damaged vessel wall.

**674. transit time**

The period that elapses as food travels from the mouth, through the digestive tract, and is expelled as waste.

**675. ulcerative**

Of an ulcer.

**676. unstirred water layer**

Region near the intestinal mucosa where water molecules remain nearly stationary.

**677. vegetarian**

A person who does not eat meat products.

**678. vein**

Vessel that carries blood to the heart.

**679. villikinin**

A mucosal hormone that causes villi to move.

## 680.  villus

Vascular tuft.

# Metabolism

### 681. acetate

A salt or ester of acetic acid.

### 682. acetone

A ketone found in blood and urine when the body is metabolizing excess fat.

### 683. acetyl-CoA

Metabolite from various kinds of molecules that is metabolized via the Krebs cycle.

### 684. adenosine triphosphate (ATP)

The body's main energy storage molecule.

### 685. aerobic

With oxygen.

### 686. aerobic system

Metabolic pathway that produces energy from amino acids, glucose and fatty acids and transfers hydrogen to oxygen.

### 687. alcohol dehydrogenase

An enzyme that metabolizes ethanol to acetaldehyde in liver cells.

### 688. alcoholism

Disease of repetitive, excessive alcohol intake, which almost always leads to severe problems in daily living.

### 689. anabolic

Of anabolism.

### 690. anabolism

Synthetic, energy using process.

**691. anaerobic**

Lacking oxygen.

**692. antidiuretic hormone**

A hormone released from the pituitary gland that causes the kidneys to reabsorb water into the blood.

**693. beta oxidation**

Metabolic pathway that oxidizes fatty acids.

**694. beta reduction**

Metabolic pathway that synthesizes fatty acids.

**695. brown fat**

Fat with a high energy content deposited around organs in newborn infants.

**696. catabolic**

Of catabolism.

**697. catabolism**

Breakdown of molecules that makes energy available.

**698. chemiosmotic theory**

Explanation of how energy is captured in mitochondria.

**699. congener**

One of many substances in alcoholic beverages that give a beverage its flavor and behavioral effects.

**700. Cori cycle**

Metabolic pathway in which lactic acid moves from muscles to the liver and glucose moves from the liver to muscles.

**701. creatine phosphate**

A molecule that accounts for limited energy storage in muscle.

**702. creatinine**

A metaboic product of creatine excreted at a constant rate in urine.

**703 deamination**

Removal of an amino group.

**704. drink (alcoholic)**

Quantity of alcoholic beverage that supplies 0.5 oz. ethanol; approximately 1 oz hard liquor, 4 oz wine, or 12 oz. beer.

**705. drug**

A substance that can modify body functions or behavior.

**706. electron transport system**

Enzymes and coenzymes in cristae of mitochondria that move electrons from substrates to oxygen.

**707. endergonic**

Requiring energy, as in a chemical reaction.

**708. energy metabolism**

All reactions that take place during the body's intake and use of food.

**709. euphoria**

A feeling of exuberant well-being achieved by some through the use of drugs.

**710. exergonic**

Releasing energy, as in a chemical reaction.

**711. fasting**

The deliberate refusal to eat.

**712. fatty liver**

Accumulation of fat in liver tissue seen in early stages of liver disease, especially in alcoholism and malnutrition.

**713. fermentation**

Metabolism of carbohydrate to alcohol and other substances in the absence of atmospheric oxygen.

**714. fibrosis**

Replacement of normal cells with fibrous connective tissue as the liver deteriorates as in alcoholism and hepatitis.

**715. flavin adenine dinucleotide (FAD)**

A coenzyme that carries hydrogen.

**716. gluconeogenesis**

Metabolic pathway that makes glucose from noncarbohydrate substances.

**717. glucose sparing**

Metabolism of fats by many cells that conserves glucose in blood for transport to cells that cannot metabolize fats.

**718. glycogenesis**

Metabolic pathway for glycogen synthesis.

**719. glycogenolysis**

Metabolic pathway for glycogen breakdown.

**720. glycolysis**

Metabolic pathway for breakdown of glucose to pyruvic acid.

**721. guanidine triphosphate (GTP)**

An energy storage molecule.

**722. half-life**

The amount of time it takes for half of a substance to be eliminated from the body.

**723. intermediate**

A molecule produced within a metabolic pathway.

**724. ketoacidosis**

A dangerous buildup of acids in the blood that sometimes seen in inadequately treated diabetes.

**725. ketone**

An organic compound produced during the oxidation of fatty acids.

**726. ketone body**

Acidic molecule that remains from incomplete metabolism of fatty acids.

**727. ketosis**

Accumulation of ketone bodies in blood and urine.

**728. Krebs cycle**

Metabolic pathway that oxidizes acetyl-CoA; citric acid cycle; tricarboxylic acid cycle.

**729. lactate**

Temporary product of anaerobic glucose metabolism.

**730. metabolic water**

Water released from the oxidation of foodstuffs.

**731. metabolism**

All chemical reactions in a living organism.

**732. mitochondrion**

An organelle that contains enzymes for oxidative and energy-capturing processes.

**733. myokinase**

An enzyme that makes ATP and AMP from 2 molecules of ADP in muscle tissue.

**734. narcotic**

A substance that impairs response to stimuli, causes sleep, and causes addiction.

**735. nicotinamide adenine dinucleotide (NAD)**

A coenzyme that transports hydrogen atoms or electrons in oxidation-reduction reactions.

**736. nitrogen balance**

The state in which nitrogen entering the body equals nitrogen leaving it.

**737. oxidative phosphorylation**

Capture of energy in ATP during oxidative metabolism.

**738. oxygen debt**

The shortage of oxygen during strenuous exercise because bloo can't bring oxygen to the muscles fast enough.

**739. pentose phosphate pathway**

Metabolic pathway that produces five-carbon sugars and reduced NADP.

**740. phosphocreatine**

An energy storage molecule found in muscle.

**741. phosphorylation**

Binding of a phosphate group to a molecule.

**742. proof**

A measure of the alcohol content of liquor; equal to two times the percent of alchol in the liquor.

**743. pyruvate**

A salt of pyruvic acid.

**744. respiratory quotient (RQ)**

Ratio of carbon dioxide released to oxygen consumed.

**745. retinopathy**

Hemorrhage of retinal capillaries, which occurs in many diabetics.

**746. transamination**

Transfer of an amino group from one molecule to another.

**747. turnover**

Breakdown and resynthesis of a substance.

**748. urea**

Product created by the liver from ammonia and carbon dioxide.

**749. urea cycle**

Metabolic pathway that synthesizes urea.

**750. xanthine**

A purine that inhibits cAMP breakdown.

# Regulation of Metabolism

**751. basal metabolic rate (BMR)**

Amount of energy used to maintain life in an awake, resting individual.

**752. basal metabolism**

The process of using energy from nutrients to maintain life in an awake, resting state.

**753. biofeedback**

Use of signals about levels of autonomic processes to control those processes.

**754. body mass index (BMI)**

Body weight (kg) divided by body height (m).

**755. calorimetry**

The measurement of energy in terms of heat.

**756. CCK-PZ (cholecystokinin-pancreozymin)**

An enteric hormone that stimulates the gallbladder to release bile and the pancreas to secrete enzymes.

**757. core body temperature**

Temperature deep within the body.

**758. coupled reaction**

The simultaneous occurrence of two chemical reactions, one of which supplies energy for the other.

**759. cross-matching**

Comparison of donor and prospective recipient bloods to detect possibilities of agglutination.

**760. diabetes mellitus**

A disorder due to lack or inactivity of insulin that allows glucose to accumulate in the blood and urine.

## 761. direct calorimetry

The measurement of energy in an organic substance by measuring heat given off during burning.

## 762. exogenous

Originating outside the body.

## 763. fasting hypoglycemia

Drop in blood glucose after 8 hour or longer fast.

## 764. frame size

Relative size of bones and musculature for a given height.

## 765. futile cycle

A metabolic cycle that expends energy without doing useful work.

## 766. glycosuria

Presence of glucose in the urine.

## 767. growth hormone-hypothalamic mechanism

A metabolic regulatory mechanism involving pituitary-related hormones.

## 768. hyperthermia

An abnormally high body temperature.

## 769. hypothermia

An abnormally low body temperature.

## 770. indirect calorimetry

The measurement of energy in an organic substance by measuring oxygen needed to cause complete burning.

## 771. insulin-dependent diabetes

Disorder of blood glucose regulation with early onset and requiring treatment with insulin.

**772. insulin-glucagon mechanism**

A mechanism that helps to regulate metabolism, especially I blood glucose.

**773. metabolic rate**

Rate at which nutrients are oxidized.

**774. noninsulin-dependent diabetes**

Disorder of blood glucose regulation with adult onset and usually treatable with diet and hypoglycemics.

**775. postabsorptive**

Related to metabolism after food from a meal is completely absorbed.

**776. pyrogen**

A substance that causes body temperature to increase.

**777. reactive hypoglycemia**

Drop in blood glucose with epinephrine release a few hours after a meal.

**778. resting metabolic rate (RMR)**

Energy output of the body at rest after fasting less than **12 hours.**

**779. satiety center**

A neural center in the hypothalamus that regulates food intake.

**780. shuttling**

Moving back and forth as between two processes.

**781. specific dynamic activity**

Thermogenesis induced by food eaten; energy used by the body to process food.

**782. thermogenesis**

Heat generation; in nutrition, the amount of energy the body is expending.

**783. thyroid gland**

A gland in the throat that produces metabolism regulating hormones.

**784. thyroid-stimulating hormone (TSH)**

A hormone that stimulates hormone secretion by the thyroid gland.

**785. uncoupling**

The disruption of a coupled reaction so that one reaction releases energy and the other fails to occur.

**786. white fat**

Fat cells that store fat and release molecules that many cells can metabolize for energy to do work.

# Weight Management / Eating Disorders

**787. adipose**

Pertaining to fat.

**788. anorexia**

Lack of appetite.

**789. anorexia nervosa**

Extreme self-starvation often seen in young women.

**790. appetite**

Desire to eat.

**791. bariatrics**

A field of science concerned with controlling body weight.

**792. behavior modification**

A set of procedures that can be helpful in changing certain activities, including eating disorders.

**793. binge eating**

Consumption of rich foods in large quantities over short periods of time.

**794. bulimia (bulemia)**

Recurrent binge eating, often followed by self-induced vomiting.

**795. bulk producers**

Substances containing dietary fiber that create a feeling of fullness by absorbing liquid in the stomach.

**796. carbohydrate-craving obesity**

Excessive body weight caused by a persistent desire for sugars and starches.

## 797. cathartic (purgative)

Laxative.

## 798. cellulite

Fat made lumpy by connective tissue, sometimes erroneously thought to differ from other fat.

## 799. emetic

Agent that induces vomiting.

## 800. external cue theory

Theory that people eat in response to time of day or sight of food and not from internal cues.

## 801. fat cell theory

Theory that overfeeding infants and children increases fat cell numbers and increases the likelihood of obesity.

## 802. fatfold test

Measure of body fatness by determining thickness of a fold of fat using calipers; skinfold test.

## 803. food diary

Record of kinds and amounts of food eaten.

## 804. food exchange system

A procedure used in some diet plans, based on average nutritional values rather than the counting of Calories.

## 805. glucostatic theory of hunger regulation

A theory asserting that changes in the blood glucose level determine when a person eats.

## 806. human chorionic gonadotropin

A hormone secreted by the placenta erroneously believed to stimulate breakdown of fat.

## 807. hunger

A sensation normally associated with the physiological need to eat.

### 808. hyperplastic obesity

Obesity associated with increased numbers of fat cells.

### 809. hypertrophic obesity

Obesity associated with increased size of fat cells.

### 810. hypothalamus

A portion of the brain that integrates signals about blood glucose level, body temperature, hunger, and satiety.

### 811. lipostatic theory of hunger regulation

A theory asserting that depletion of body fat stores causes a person to eat.

### 812. malnutrition

Ill health caused by an inadequate diet.

### 813. marasmus

Malnutrition to the degree of near-starvation.

### 814. mild obesity

The condition of weighing twenty to forty percent more than one's ideal weight.

### 815. moderate obesity

The condition of weighing forty-one to one hundred percent more than one's ideal weight.

### 816. obesity

Excessive body fatness, usually more than 20 percent above weight specified in life insurance tables.

### 817. overweight

Body weight 10 percent above weight specified in life insurance tables.

### 818. purinergic theory of hunger regulation

A theory asserting that purines circulating in blood determine eating behavior.

**819. ratchet effect**

Weight loss without exercise followed by greater weight gain; body fat increases and caloric needs decrease.

**820. set point**

Point at which a body process is at optimum level; weight below which gain occurs and above which loss occurs.

**821. severe obesity**

The condition of weighing more than twice one's ideal weight.

**822. total parental nutrition (TPN)**

Process of giving all required nutrients by a route other than the digestive tract.

**823. underweight**

Body weight 10 percent below weight specified in life insurance tables.

# Food Safety and Labeling

**824. additive**

A substance not naturally found in food.

**825. Ames test**

A test that uses bacteria to identify agents that cause mutations and that might be carcinogens.

**826. anticaking agent**

A substance added to a food to keep it free flowing.

**827. antimicrobial agent**

Any substance that inhibits bacterial growth.

**828. antioxidant**

A substance added to a food to retard oxidation.

**829. arable**

In reference to land, capable of being plowed (usually for growing food).

**830. aspartame**

An artificial sweetener composed of amino acids.

**831. bleach**

A substance added to whiten a food such as cheese or flour.

**832. botulism**

A severe form of food poisoning caused by botulinum toxin from a bacterium.

**833. carcinogen**

An agent that initiates events leading to cancer.

**834. carcinogenesis**

The development of cancer.

**835. carcinogenic**

Cancer-causing.

**836. coloring agent**

A substance added to a food to give it a more appealing color.

**837. cyclamate**

An artificial sweetener used in Canada but banned in the United States.

**838. D-amino acid**

Mirror image of natural L-amino acid, which body enzyme cannot metabolize.

**839. Delaney clause**

A law that prevents adding to foods any substance known to cause cancer in animals or humans at any dosage.

**840. diketopiperazine**

Breakdown product of aspartame.

**841. dose-response relationship**

A relationship between how much of a substance is given and the level of its effects.

**842. emulsifier**

A substance that keeps components of a food bound.

**843. enterotoxin**

Poison in the intestinal tract that has been produced by bacteria in food.

**844. excision enzyme**

Enzyme that removes defective segments from a DNA molecule.

**845. expiration date**

The latest date that a particular package of
food can be consumed safely.

**846. flavoring agent**

A substance added to a food to enhance its taste.

**847. food additives**

Any matter that becomes a part of, or affects the
characteristics of, a food product.

**848. food consumption survey**

A study of kinds and amounts of food people consume compared
with standards such as RDAs.

**849. foodborne infection**

Any adverse condition caused by food that has been
contaminated by a substantial number of living organisms.

**850. frame shift mutation**

An addition or deletion of one or more bases in DNA such
that the sequence of codons is altered.

**851. freshness date**

The latest date on which a particular package of food,
usually baked goods, will have its normal taste.

**852. fungicide**

A substance that kills fungi and can cause birth defects and
other toxic effects if present in food.

**853. GRAS list**

A list of food additives generally recognized as safe.

**854. halogen**

An atom such as chlorine, fluorine, bromine, or iodine.

**855. hazard**

A danger.

**856.** **heavy metal**

Element with high atomic weight such as lead or mercury that denatures proteins and causes other toxic effects.

**857.** **herbicide**

A substance that kills weeds and can act as a neurotoxin or carcinogen if present in food.

**858.** **high fructose corn syrup (HFCS)**

A commercially-produced sugar that is made sweeter than most sugars through the use of certain enzymes.

**859.** **humectant**

A substance added to a food to help it retain moisture.

**860.** **indirect additive**

A substance that enters food during processing, storage, or other operations prior to consumption.

**861.** **infant mortality rate**

Number of deaths during first year of life per 1000 live born infants.

**862.** **insecticide**

A substance that kills insects and can act as a neurotoxin or carcinogen; some can accumulate in tissues.

**863.** **intentional additive**

A substance such as a dye or a nutrient purposely added to a food.

**864.** **L-sugar**

Mirror image of natural D-sugar, which body enzymes cannot metabolize.

**865.** **leavening agent**

A substance added to a food to give it a lighter texture.

**866.** **low-birth-weight baby**

Infant that ways less than 2500 grams at birth.

**867. margin of safety**

Difference between concentration of a substance normally present and the concentration that produces toxic effects.

**868. mutagenesis**

The production of mutations.

**869. neutralizing agent**

A substance added to a food to control variation in acidity or alkalinity.

**870. nitrite**

A nitrogenous salt used as a preservative, especially to prevent botulism.

**871. nitrosamine**

A carcinogen formed in the stomach from nitrites and amines.

**872. nutrition status survey**

A study to evaluate the nutritional status of a population from case histories, physical exams, and lab tests.

**873. organic halogen**

An organic molecule with one or more halogen atoms attached.

**874. pack date**

The day upon which a particular can or other package of food was manufactured.

**875. phenylketonuria**

A hereditary disorder in which the amino acid tyrosine cannot be metabolized and toxic phenylketones accumulate.

**876. picowave**

A general term for a very small amount of radiation suitable for preventing food spoilage.

**877. point mutation**

A change in a single base in DNA.

**878. polychlorinated biphenyl**

A synthetic substance from electrical equipment that now contaminates fatty tissues of humans and other animals.

**879. preservative**

A substance added to a food to prevent spoilage.

**880. quantitative risk assessment**

An estimate of how much damage an agent might cause.

**881. repair enzyme**

Enzyme that helps to synthesize new DNA to replace defective segments removed.

**882. restoration**

The practice of adding nutrients to food products to compensate for nutrients lost during processing.

**883. risk assessment**

An estimate of whether or not an agent causes damage.

**884. rodenticide**

A substance that kills rodents and can act as anticoagulant, or cause heart failure or metabolic disorders.

**885. saccharin**

An artificial sweetener used in the United States but banned in Canada.

**886. stabilizer**

A substance that maintains texture of a food.

**887. sulfite**

Sulfur-based substances that are widely used by the food industry as antioxidants and preservatives.

**888. toxicity**

Ability of a substance to cause harm to a living thing.

### 889. unique radiolytic product (URP)

An apparently harmless molecule formed when food is irradiated.

# Nutrition at Different Life Stages

**890. adolescence**

Period from the onset of puberty and adulthood.

**891. aging**

Process of growing old.

**892. allergy**

A condition characterized by symptoms that are reaction to a substance to which the body has become sensitized.

**893. amniotic fluid**

Liquid surrounding the fetus in utero.

**894. amniotic sac**

Baglike structure in the uterus in which the fetus floats.

**895. antigen**

A foreign substance that brings about the formation of antibodies or inflammation.

**896. aseptic technique**

Laboratory procedure that prevents unwanted microorganisms from contaminating a substance.

**897. asymptomatic**

Lacking effects that can be noticed by the patient.

**898. athletes' amenorrhea**

Failure of female athlete to menstruate.

**899. athletes' anemia**

Anemia seen in athletes that has no known cause.

**900. athletic osteoporosis**

Bone loss in athletes, especially female runners with anorexia.

**901. beikost**

Weaning food.

**902. bifidus factor**

Substance in colostrum and breast milk that fosters growth of desirable intestinal bacteria.

**903. bonding**

Formation of a special, close association as between mother and infant.

**904. cardiac index**

Cardiac output per square meter of body surface.

**905. cardiac output**

Blood volume pumped per minute; equals stroke volume times heart rate.

**906. casein (sodium caseinate)**

Main protein in cow's milk.

**907. colostrum**

Fluid secreted from the breasts for the first few days after delivery.

**908. condensed milk**

Evaporated milk to which sugar has been added.

**909. convergence**

Coming together.

**910. critical period**

A developmental period between fertilization and implantation during which the dividing zygote is very vulnerable.

**911. eclampsia**

Convulsions and coma in severe toxemia, usually seen shortly before or after birth.

**912. embryo**

An infant during the second to eighth weeks of development.

**913. epiphysis**

End segment of a long bone that has a thin area of active bone growth in young people.

**914. estrogen replacement**

A therapy sometimes used to prevent or manage osteoporosis.

**915. evaporated milk**

Milk decreased in volume by half by evaporation of water.

**916. evaporated milk formula**

Infant formula made from evaporated milk.

**917. fetal alcohol syndrome (FAS)**

Mental and physical retardation in a child born to a mother who consumed an excess of alcohol during pregnancy.

**918. fetus**

An infant from the ninth week of development to birth.

**919. fortified**

Food to which nutrients have been added, such as milk with added vitamins A and D.

**920. glycogen loading**

Manipulation of carbohydrates in diet to cause muscles to store maximum amounts of glycogen.

**921. homogenized milk**

Milk treated with heat under pressure that breaks fat droplets into small particles that remain suspended.

### 922. hyperactivity syndrome

A set of symptoms including short attention span and impulsive behaviors.

### 923. hyperplasia

An increase in cell number.

### 924. implantation

Stage at which a fertilized egg embeds itself in the wall of the uterus and begins to develop.

### 925. infancy

The period of time from 1 month to 2 years of age.

### 926. lactalbumin

Main protein in human milk.

### 927. lactation

Synthesis and secretion of milk.

### 928. lactiferous

Making or conveying milk.

### 929. life expectancy

The average number of years of life for members of a population at a given age.

### 930. life span

The maximum length of the life for a member of a given species.

### 931. lipofuscin

Pigment associated with aging.

### 932. mammary gland

Gland that synthesizes and secretes milk.

**933. menarche**

Developmental stage at which menstruation begins.

**934. milk anemia**

Anemia due to dietary iron deficiency from prolonged diet of mainly milk without iron rich foods.

**935. mitochondria**

Intracellular organelles that contain enzymes responsible for oxidative metabolism.

**936. neonatal period**

The period of time from birth to one month of age.

**937. neonate**

A newborn infant.

**938. neuroglial**

Related to supporting cells of the nervous system.

**939. parasympatholytic**

Concerning substances that block or counteract sympathetic signals.

**940. parturition**

Childbirth.

**941. pasteurized milk**

Milk treated with sufficient heat to reduce number of bacteria, including killing pathogens that might be present.

**942. pica**

A craving for a nonnutritive substance such as starch or clay.

**943. placenta**

Structure attached to the uterine wall that provides nutrients and removes wastes for a developing fetus.

**944. powdered milk**

Solids remaining when milk is completely dehydrated.

**945. preeclampsia**

Eclampsia-like symptoms seen during pregnancy that may lead to eclampsia.

**946. pregnancy-induced hypertension**

Edema, hypertension, and kidney disease seen in pregnancy; toxemia.

**947. premature**

Born before expected time but of normal size for gestational age.

**948. puberty**

Period during which sexual maturation occurs.

**949. renal solute load**

Concentration of dissolved substances in urine that result from diet, especially breast milk or infant formula.

**950. salicylate**

Substance such as aspirin and yellow dye (tartrazine); sometimes cause allergies.

**951. small for gestational age**

Small birth size for the length of time under development.

**952. superoxide dismutase**

An antioxidant enzyme fraudulently sold to counteract aging.

**953. symptomatic**

Producing effects noticed by the patient.

**954. thymus**

An organ that helps in the maturation of T cells, and is much smaller in elderly people than in young adults.

### 955. urinary incontinence

The inability to control the muscle that controls urination.

### 956. uterus

The womb.

### 957. vital capacity

The maximum volume of gas that can be inhaled or exhaled.

### 958. whole milk

Milk with nothing added or removed; legally must contain at least 3.25% fat and 8.25% nonfat milk solids.

# Index

| | | | |
|---|---|---|---|
| diabetes mellitus | 75 | erythocyte | 35 |
| diarrhea | 56 | erythrocyte | 46 |
| diastole | 45 | erythrocyte protoporphyrin | 46 |
| diet record | 1 | esophageal | 57 |
| dietary fiber | 15 | esophagus | 58 |
| dietary goals | 1 | essential amino acid | 27 |
| dietary history | 2 | essential fatty acid | 20 |
| dietary recall | 2 | essential nutrient | 2 |
| digestibility (of protein) | 26 | estrogen | 20 |
| digestion | 56 | estrogen replacement | 92 |
| diketopiperazine | 84 | euphoria | 70 |
| dipeptidase | 26 | evaporated milk | 92 |
| dipeptide | 27 | evaporated milk formula | 92 |
| direct calorimetry | 76 | excision enzyme | 84 |
| disaccharide | 15 | exergonic | 70 |
| diuretic | 45 | exogenous | 76 |
| diverticulitis | 56 | exogenous nitrogen | 27 |
| diverticulosis | 56 | expiration date | 85 |
| dose-response relationship | 84 | external cue theory | 80 |
| double blind | 2 | extracellular | 46 |
| drink (alcoholic) | 70 | facilitated diffusion | 58 |
| drug | 70 | fasting | 70 |
| duodenal | 57 | fasting hypoglycemia | 76 |
| duodenum | 57 | fat | 20 |
| dysentery | 57 | fat cell theory | 80 |
| eclampsia | 92 | fat-soluble vitamins | 35 |
| edema | 57 | fatfold test | 80 |
| electrolyte | 45 | fatty acid | 20 |
| electron | 8 | fatty liver | 70 |
| electron transport system | 70 | feces | 58 |
| element | 8 | feedback system | 58 |
| embolus | 57 | fermentation | 71 |
| embryo | 92 | ferric ion | 46 |
| emetic | 80 | ferritin | 46 |
| emulsification | 20 | ferrous ion | 46 |
| emulsifier | 84 | fetal alcohol syndrome (FAS) | 92 |
| emulsify | 20 | fetus | 92 |
| enamel | 35 | fiber | 15 |
| endergonic | 70 | fibrin | 27 |
| endocrine glands | 57 | fibrinogen | 27 |
| endogenous nitrogen | 27 | fibrocystic breast disease | 36 |
| endogenous opiate | 57 | fibrosis | 71 |
| endogenous protein | 27 | filtration | 58 |
| endorphin | 27 | flavin adenine dinucleotide (FAD) | 71 |
| energy metabolism | 70 | flavoring agent | 85 |
| enkephalin | 27 | fluid regulation | 46 |
| enriched food | 2 | fluorapatite | 46 |
| enterogastric reflex | 57 | fluorosis | 46 |
| enterogastrone | 57 | folacin | 36 |
| enterohepatic circulation | 20 | follicle | 36 |
| enterokinase | 27 | follicular hyperkeratosis | 36 |
| enterotoxin | 84 | fontanel | 36 |
| enzyme | 8 | food | 2 |
| epidemiology | 2 | food additives | 85 |
| epiglottis | 57 | food composition tables | 2 |
| epinephrine | 20 | food consumption survey | 85 |
| epiphysis | 92 | food diary | 80 |
| epithelial cell | 35 | food disappearance study | 2 |
| epithelium | 35 | food exchange system | 80 |
| ergocalciferol | 35 | food fortification | 36 |

| | | | |
|---|---|---|---|
| hypoglycemia | 16 | lactation | 93 |
| hypoglycemic | 16 | lacteal | 61 |
| hyposmotic | 10 | lactiferous | 93 |
| hypothalamus | 81 | lacto-ovo-vegetarian | 28 |
| hypothermia | 76 | lactose | 10 |
| hypotonic | 10 | lactose intolerance | 10 |
| hypoxia | 60 | lamina propria | 61 |
| ileostomy | 60 | latent | 61 |
| ileum | 60 | lean tissue | 3 |
| immune system | 3 | leavening agent | 86 |
| immunity | 3 | lecithin | 21 |
| implantation | 93 | lesion | 61 |
| indirect additive | 86 | lethal | 61 |
| indirect calorimetry | 76 | leukocyte ferritin | 48 |
| infancy | 93 | life expectancy | 93 |
| infant mortality rate | 86 | life span | 93 |
| infarct | 60 | ligand | 11 |
| insecticide | 86 | lignin | 16 |
| insensible | 48 | limiting amino acid | 28 |
| insulin | 16 | lingual | 61 |
| insulin shock | 16 | lipase | 21 |
| insulin-dependent diabetes | 76 | lipid | 21 |
| insulin-glucagon mechanism | 77 | lipofuscin | 93 |
| intentional additive | 86 | lipophilic | 21 |
| intermediate | 71 | lipophobic | 21 |
| intermittent claudication | 37 | lipoprotein | 21 |
| international unit | 37 | lipoprotein lipase | 21 |
| intestinal | 60 | lipostatic theory of hunger | |
| intestinal flora | 60 | regulation | 81 |
| intracellular | 48 | liver | 61 |
| intravenous | 60 | longitudinal study | 3 |
| intrinsic factor (IF) | 37 | low density lipoprotein (LDL) | 21 |
| ion | 10 | low-birth-weight baby | 86 |
| ionic bond | 10 | lymph | 61 |
| iron overload | 48 | lymphatic system | 61 |
| ischemia | 60 | lysosome | 38 |
| ischemic heart disease | 61 | macrobiotic diet | 28 |
| islet of Langerhans | 16 | macromolecule | 11 |
| isomer | 10 | major mineral | 48 |
| isosmotic | 10 | malnutrition | 81 |
| isotonic | 10 | maltase | 16 |
| isotope | 10 | maltose | 11 |
| jaundice | 38 | mammary gland | 93 |
| jejunum | 61 | marasmus | 81 |
| kelp | 38 | margin of safety | 87 |
| keratin | 38 | meat replacement | 28 |
| keratomalacia | 38 | meat-fish-poultry (MFP) factor | 48 |
| kernicterus | 38 | megadose | 38 |
| Keshan disease | 48 | melanin | 29 |
| ketoacidosis | 72 | menadione | 38 |
| ketone | 72 | menarche | 94 |
| ketone body | 72 | mesentery | 62 |
| ketosis | 72 | metabolic acidosis | 48 |
| kilocalorie | 3 | metabolic alkalosis | 48 |
| Krebs cycle | 72 | metabolic nitrogen | 29 |
| kwashiorkor | 28 | metabolic rate | 77 |
| L-sugar | 86 | metabolic water | 72 |
| lactalbumin | 93 | metabolism | 72 |
| lactase | 16 | metalloenzyme | 48 |
| lactate | 72 | metallothionine | 49 |